AF885548

How to live to be 200 years old

Living Well, Living Long: Mastering Tips for a Happy, Healthy, Extended Life and Better Longevity

by

Zafer Roback

Prologue

In a time when healthier, longer lives seem to be out of reach, this book is a light in the darkness and a source of practical advice. The author, Zafer Roback, is not only a researcher but he has spent his whole life trying to figure out how to live long and happy, not just how to spend more years on the planet but how to make those years meaningful and worth living. By integrating the body, mind, and spirit as individual components of health, Roback provides readers with a strong and comprehensive approach to well-being.

From his research and personal exploration in his lifetime, he incorporates scientific knowledge, realistic knowledge, and eternal knowledge to guide the reader through the process of achieving great health and well-being. May this book serve as your compass that will navigation you through today's complex world full of enticements and diversions. Take the author's advice to heart and learn how to not only live longer, but live better.

In this book you will find a way through the maze of the contemporary world with ever increasing number of seductions and distractions. Follow the words of the author, and discover how to live not only longer, but to live better, writes the author. Start this amazing journey and learn what it means to live long – not by the number of years but by the quality and value of the life we lead. May this book be your friend, guide, and inspiration for leading a good life. In this prologue, life longevity and wellness are presented as the main subjects in the book as well as the author's professional background and the encompassing nature of the book. It also points to the positive change that is possible in one's life when one reads the content of the book and follows the guidelines therein.

Table of Contents

Prologue *4*

Dedication.. *8*

Acknowledgement... *9*

Chapter 1: Dangers of Drugs and Alcohol *11*

Chapter 2: Building the Self-Reliance and Leadership *24*

Chapter 3: Establishing the Healthy Routine *47*

Chapter 4: Maintaining the Physical and Mental Health *67*

Conclusion.. *88*

Book Review Call.. *94*

Dedication

I dedicated this book to my loving wife Carolyn Ann Roback, who supported me in every step of life and guide me to take a necessary action where it is needed. Without her unwavering encouragement, this work would not have been possible.

Acknowledgement

My sincere gratitude to my partner and best friend Graham Norris, for the valuable contribution as an editor and proof-reader. His supervision and suggestions have been a great help in the making of this book and his appreciation for details makes him a handy man to have around.

I also wish to express my profound thanks to a good friend Stan Bass for the excellent job he has done in the professional photography for this book. His creativity, and mastery in the work has been an asset and instrumental to his success.

In this regard, I would like to express my sincere appreciation to the following persons and institutions. Your efforts in participation either directly or via providing support of various forms have been incredibly useful and I want to thank you for the hard work, time and effort you have invested in this project.

Chapter 1: Dangers of Drugs and Alcohol

The moment you were born, you started dying. A good many babies do die at birth. Why? Because of their parents. Their parents did not take care of themselves. Many parents are still babies themselves. Through their teen years until they become twenty-one years old. It would be best if you strived to become an older adult as soon as possible. Think as if you (the kid) are in charge of your life.

You can reach your "one hundred" birthday easily. You are what you eat, what you drink, what you smoke. At the end of the day, what have you accomplished? Not a thing!!! At age 15 or so, you start following your friend's ways. "They drink alcohol, and you drink alcohol." "They smoke cigarettes, you smoke cigarettes."

"They rob banks, you rob banks," "They speed drive the car, you speed drive the car." They are your leaders, so they must be right. NO! You should grow up and become a leader. You can live to be 100 years old or so. They were your leaders, and now they are six feet underground, starting at age 15 or so, because of bad habits.

What you put in your mouth starts the ball rolling. That one bite of food goes through the same process all foods undergo. Medicines, drugs, and liquids—whiskey, beer, cigarettes—go through the same pathway to the toilet.

Regardless of your intention, the good, the bad, and the ugly end in the toilet. What you consume is equally important as your body and brain work together. What you put in your body through your mouth or veins is especially important, and what you put into your bloodstream is also especially important.

What you put in your mouth goes into

your body and affects your body, brain, and longevity. Be very careful of what you put between those lips. Some of the results are:

A) Your hips become large.

B) Your eyes become weak.

C) Your brain becomes dull.

D) Your body becomes ugly.

E) Your mouth will have a very, very bad smell/odor

F) Your teeth will be seen by everyone you talk to or smile. The color will be black, yellow, or green teeth, the worst of all missing teeth.

I know that I talk about drinking a lot, sorry!! But I've seen what happens. I can only save a few people and lives by speaking and writing about it. Alcohol affects all people the same. Not able to walk in a straight line. Not able to talk or control themselves. Your life is shorter by 25 years to 50 years because of drinking. Your wife or your girlfriend or your husband or boyfriend are all affected to a degree if you drink. Even your children are affected.

Drinking alcohol is bad for you regardless of how little you drink or how much you drink. You can have a lot more fun, plus keep a lot of money in your pocket to spend on your kids and wife. My friends, embarking on the path of longevity and wellness is a journey that demands courage and commitment. While peer pressure may seem daunting, remember that staying true to your values is not just a choice but a powerful act of self-empowerment that will reward you tenfold in the long run.

As adolescents, we naturally crave independence and recognition from our peers. However, we must be wary of false ideas of acceptance that come at the cost of our well-being. Toxic influences like drugs and alcohol may provide fleeting pleasure, yet they take a heavy toll on the mind and body if indulged. Don't let dubious claims of "just having fun" or "fitting in" distract you from your greater purpose.

You all have so much to unlock and unleash in yourselves and your lives: gifts, passions, friends, and so much more. Will poison assist you in this process of development? Or will it hinder your ability to achieve your best self by clouding your mind, draining your energy, and negatively impacting your future health? These are questions that one has to think about.

Surrounded by friends who encourage your well-being and support your decision to stand up for what is right, it becomes increasingly easier to make the right decisions for your health and well-being every day. It is advisable to set some time for such people who make you perform your best during the activities you two engage in, the conversations you have, and the things you do for each other.

Avoid the company of those who would seek to erode your values for the sake of immediate gratification or peer pressure. O' my friends, this 'little' thing is Quite impressive and extraordinary: You are the naive sculptors of reality. It requires courage to listen to the positive guiding spirit within oneself, especially when every negative sign from the outside world is against you.

Adhere to spending time and energy on building and maintaining supporting relations and pursuits that promote the well-being of the physical body, mind, and environment. True happiness defines a mature life attentive to virtue, not fake happiness that resides in sinful indulgence or hypocrisy.

Do not forget that there will still be much growth, ideas, and modes of serving your fellow people in the future. Step up and strive for the best self, and never allow anything to hinder the full shining of the real you. Endeavor strength as a virtue assures that everything an individual requires to persevere and triumph, even under challenging circumstances, is achievable.

I know that you have the potential for wisdom and bravery. Well, now you have surpassed the knowledge and run – and glow! Not now; go and walk in the sunshine! Live passionately how you envision, and ink it into your reality. Even if the journey is unclear, it is still important to follow your values, and integrity will not do you wrong.

The words embodied in this design assert that one must find the courage within oneself when external influences attempt to push one in a specific direction. True north is the truth about yourself that only you understand; others may not see it and rightly tend to it. My dear, still believe in the voice inside you whispering about health, purpose, and integrity. This means that there is no reason to doubt that you can create the bright future you have in mind.

To be sure, difficulties will never be far, but each day you refuse temptation and feed your soul sufficiently, the two possibilities—health and happiness in old age draw nearer. As we know, there is often an enormous temptation for immediate satisfaction, but we do not live for contingents but for gains. Complex unknowns can be parsed into simple terms: Take a breath and commit to any decision that honors your soul. Gradually change your room to put in what you think is worthy and motivating.

Cherish for each to release what binds them to less than their potential. In this reference, change every situation into a positive one that leads to growth. To rein in your emotions and not over-excite in essential situations, remember that you do not walk this path alone. Do not hesitate to turn to someone and find support from a friend during difficult periods, even if it is just in the form of a listening ear and encouragement.

As we saw earlier, there is often reciprocity in these interactions; for example, when the favor is due, others help us similarly when we need it. But with the knowledge of our strong wall and the strength of his gentle heart, we could conquer all of our fears.

Therefore, let there be hope, my dear friend; let your soul light up, for you can also be a shining light to others. It will be a great pleasure to serve and share your examples of wellness and wisdom to make a difference in ways one cannot even imagine. If it will be too tricky, remain persistent and calm, for the journey is a blessing to both yourself and humanity. And now go for it – the day has asked for it!"

Chapter 2: Building the Self-Reliance and Leadership

Drink a soft drink, a sprite, or water. I have been to different social events, and I have been to parties where people got stinking stupid drunk. Besides being drunk, you will make an ass of yourself. Drinking will shorten your life.

Intoxicated drivers have accidents. Drunken drivers kill themselves and kill others.

Drunks have killed their whole family. Drinking affects your body and all its organs. Your kidneys try to filter everything that passes through them. Your throat, stomach, kidneys, and intestines suffer from what passes through them and your body. Your friends will try to pressure you to drink with them.

I have sat with them and with some of the most famous people in the world—the choice to drink Sprite, Coke, or water instead of alcohol. If you must drink alcohol, before you start drinking, start eating a sandwich with melted butter on two slices of bread about one hour before you start partying. Also, eat again during the party. I was in Amman, Jordan, doing a project for King Hassan's Jordanian government.

All the people doing the project, like road workers, office workers, and business people, were at the King Hussein complex. We were all having a party and having a great time, eating and drinking. There were about one hundred people there. Ten guests were at each big round table. A waiter was going around all the tables, asking at each table, "What did they want to drink?" When he came around to me, I said, "Coke." He said, "No, no, no!" I said Pepsi, and he said, "No!".

I said coffee, and he said, "No, no!"

Then he said, whiskey, wine, beer? In a loud voice, my cousin said, "My cousin does not drink; bring him what he wants. The order taker turned and ran away. In a few minutes, another gentleman came to our table and asked, "Who is the gentleman who drinks "coke?" I said, "I do."

The gentleman handed me a can of coke and said, "Do not ever drink!!! Alcohol, you will be a better person." That gentleman was King Hussein of Jordan. We became good friends, and I took his advice as well. As it was, King Hussein was also a black belt in Judo, and I am also a black belt in Judo. We worked out together in his private gym in his palace several times. On a side note, in

January 1963, I was given a full scholarship for Judo and Karate at the "University of the Cumberland" in Williamsburg, Kentucky.

I also was on the tennis team, the track team, the basketball team's trainer, and the Judo team's captain and trainer. If I had drank and smoked, I could not have done one sport, let alone the other sports. I advise you as a young person to "Stop that bad habit. Better yet, don't ever start. You will thank me someday. Do all the exercises that I have done and live to be 200 years old.

Besides being healthy, you will look great in your clothes. Your mind will be able to speak with great common sense to your mother, father, girlfriend, boys, and fellow workers. Besides not drinking, join a health club and start a workout program. If you do not know how to work out, that's no problem. The instructors at the health club will teach you how to work out the right way. This is the best thing that you can ever do for yourself.

It will be the greatest and best way to spend your money, the greatest and best way to live right, and the greatest and best way always to look great and feel great. I joined the Health Spa. John Paskill was my first instructor. He is now 92 years old and going strong. All the above can be avoided if you want to do the right thing: eat, drink, do not smoke, and get eight hours of sleep every night.

Doing as I say will help you feel better, look better, and act better. Best of all, you can live to be 200 years old. It is a great start to being a pleased person who is liked by many and loved by few. Farmers grow tobacco, that is a "No! No!" If you smoke, chew, or snort, it is a no! No! Not good. If you smoke, "your lips," "your mouth," "your throat," and "your lungs' ' are all subject to developing cancer, and you will die!!!

Besides having bad breath, yellow teeth, cancer of the throat, and the big one, you get lung cancer, kissing a person who smokes is like "licking a full ashtray." Gross!!! Be it any cigarette or cigar, you will get cancer, and you will die eventually. If you vape because it looks cool, you will die. Your lungs are for you to inhale and exhale clean air, God-given oxygen. Put oxygen in your lungs, and keep a healthy body and brain. I have been all over the world.

I have met a lot of people at different parties who drank alcohol. They made an ass of themselves before a lot of people because they drank and got drunk and did not know...when to stop. Many drunks go from a bar to home in their car. Many drunk men and drunk women have caused car accidents. Many people died, both drunk person and sober person, because of that drunk person. The body that is most affected by drinking alcohol.

The best thing is not ever to start

drinking. Alcohol affects all people in the same way. They cannot walk a straight line, think, and control themselves. First, your life is shortened by 25 to 50 years because of alcohol. Your wife, girlfriend, husband, or boyfriend are all affected if you drink. Even your children are affected by your drinking alcohol. Regardless of how little or how much you drink.

Drink coke, sprite, or water. I have been to many different social events, and I have been to parties where people got stinking stupid drunk; besides being drunk, you will make an ass of yourself and use your brain to keep your body healthy and strong and beautiful. Please do not listen to stupid people, your friends, your spouse, your parents, or your boss, because they want you to drink, smoke, take pills, get vein injections, and snort cocaine.

They are not your friend or your God. They want your money and want to be your God. Please think for yourself; do not be a party pleaser. A very dear friend of mine begged me to drink a glass of alcohol with him for three hours. The bottle had a worm in it. I said "no" about ten times. Finally, I filled a big glass of whiskey and let him and all ten of his friends watch me pour the entire glass of expensive whiskey outside in the grass.

He was a dear friend of mine, and we continued to be good friends until he died a year later. Use your brain to keep your body healthy, strong, and beautiful. Do not let stupid people or stupid friends go down the path of dying early in life. Help them, advise them, and keep them healthy and alive. You will never regret it.

The goal of true self-reliance and leadership is to have the right mindset of developing long term sustainability and not indulging in immediate pleasures. Taking proper decisions benefits your health at the same time inspire others with good examples. This principle is not limited to abstaining from alcohol and drugs only but involves a lot more. It involves the aspect of togetherness that refers to the lending of support on the mental, physical, and spiritual aspect as well as the aspect of ethics.

It is habits of work, healthy self-reliant habits on which positive self-reliant life is built. A daily regimen, which includes exercise, accustoming yourself to proper eating and engaging in activities that will help you to relax and de-stress will literally transform your existence for the better. Exercise enhances the body muscles, lifts your mood, and assists in increasing energy levels in people. It also involves discipline and diligence which are favorable characteristics for a leader.

Other important habits are regard Health eating. A healthy diet plan that is composed of fruits, vegetables, lean sources of proteins, and whole grain supplies your body with necessary nutrients for efficiency. A closer look at nutrition identifies that the elimination of refined foods and the moderation of sugar leads to reduction in disease occurrence and helps people maintain healthy body weights.

This form of relaxation entails the utilization of techniques such as meditation, and deep breathing exercises which can improve mental functioning, and stabilize the emotions. It assists you to cope with stress, attend to the important things, or make right decisions. The mentioned practices can be integrated into everyday life and help to achieve better quality of life.

A lot of people have expressed that mental resilience can be defined as the capability to regain one's ground and to keep a cheerful disposition after a struggle. It is possible to build it by practice when a person is willing and ready to change and has good impulses self-control. Personal critical awareness is all about having cognizance of strengths, weaknesses, as well as the things that may prompt a person to act in a specific manner.

It makes it possible for the holder to handle sensitive or delicate moments in the most professional and dignified manner. A growth mindset on the other hand means that one gives his or her best when faced with challenging task since the individual believes that he or she can develop his or her ability and intelligence.

Adopting this type of thinking assists in encouraging one to see the inability to achieve something as a positive event not a negative one. It fosters personal and professional growth and that is essential for leadership.

Managing emotions engages understanding and exercising control over them. Emotional regulation entails the ability to handle emotions in a way that one controls how he or she responds to situations without the influences of emotions.

Management is not about making people obey your orders; it is about helping them reach their destination. Demonstrating a positive behaviour or attitude is one of the effective ways of positive behavioural change. Whenever the endorser himself displays conduct in line with the message he conveyed to the public, people will follow him because of the confidence in what he practices.

Integrity, accountability and empathy are crucial when leading other people either in an organization, company or even in a team. Ethics refers to being honest in conduct as well as adhering to some principles. Responsibility means the manner in which, one is willing to accept responsibility for their actions and decisions, to confess their mistakes and to correct them as well. Empathy entails coming up with solutions to the problems facing or that may be of interest to other people.

In this way, people observe that you, the leader, act honestly and responsibly, making them acts motivated and encouraging them. It is thought that many people would listen and obey those who, to some extent, have custody of their welfare. Anything in life is not done single handedly.

The cultivation of the social capital entails the development of a supportive social network, which is paramount for the growth and development of any person. Aim to be around people who will motivate you and pencil in the positive people into your life calendar. Try to find those people who are successful and can share some of the tips from their practice. The global economy is very dynamic, and flexibility is key when it comes to continuous success.

Pursue this habit by obtaining intimate knowledge about the subject that one has to pursue in order to be fit for the position with updated information. This can be attained through a training program, reading, going for a workshop or even taking a new sport or any other activity.

Flexibility is the ability to receive change and be ready to go the extra mile or do things in a different way. Always welcome new changes and competition as a reason to improve. As a result, one can become relevant and ready for a shift in the different settings that may be present in one's life.

Basically, ethical decision making is one of the core principles of ethical leadership. It is a practice that entails bearing in mind the effects that your action will have on other people, as well as making decisions that are bound to strong, viable ethics. The potential benefit to the various parties is the topmost agenda of ethical leaders as opposed to a self-serving benefit.

Faced with any kind of decision, always consider the complexity of the decision and the likely outcomes it would produce. Without any doubt, turn to others and take an opportunity for a self-analysis. Ethics help in creating perfect decision and impression amongst the followers, so it is an important way of leadership.

One should always aim at being in proper health so as to be in a position to lead and bring change in societies. It is a no brainer that, you must go for a medical checkup regularly maintain, a proper diet, sleep, and exercise to maintain optimal energy and productivity. This is quite dangerous, as it can cause burnout and a reduction in leadership capabilities due to negligence of one's health.

To improve upon the health life, you need to go for preventive measures, this can be achieved by going for health check-ups to know your general health status. It does not just improve your life experience, but guarantees that you can keep on guiding other people.

Independence in the matters of finance is also one of the important features of self-sufficiency. Pruding for your financial resources means that one will be able provide his or her needs and those of a close one without applying to much pressure. Develop a personal budget and accumulate some money for the future, choosing a reasonable and wise way to act in the field of expenditure and investments.

Proper finance is indeed the key to the success of performing its goals and dreams in an individual's life. It also enables you to help other people in their time of needs thus creating the component of security and togetherness.

Selflessness is always the best form of leadership that an individual can portray. It is noble to give back to your fellow human beings, especially the needy, as this will result in many more cycles of positive giving. Give your time, donate your things and use your talents in serving the people. Not only is service an effective way to help others, but it also positively influences the life of a person who performs it since there is always a feeling of fullness received from service.

Empowering oneself and becoming a leader is a process that cannot be achieved in a short time and receiving a high-quality education. It was established that by gaining positive character, psychological hardness, role modeling, social support, personal and academic development, ethical reasoning, fitness, financial responsibility, and volunteering, a good framework for a meaningful and productive life is established. Adopt these principles and others will follow your lead, when one turns a new page in life to find strength, integrity and compassion, he/she starts the same journey for others.

Chapter 3: Establishing the Healthy Routine

Do the right thing and do not drink alcohol of any kind so you can be accepted by your friends. If you are a girl with a boyfriend who drinks and smokes, kick him to the curb if he does not stop. The same goes if you are a man and your girlfriend smokes, drinks, and says goodbye!! You will live longer and happier. Besides, alcohol is bad for your health.

It is terrible for your body, and drinking "makes" you stupid drunk. When you drink and drive home, you will have an accident. You may kill yourself and your girlfriend and your kids and people in the other car. You will go to jail or an early grave, and this does ruin a lot of lives. You go to prison, or you go to the cemetery forever.

You may now think this guy knows nothing about his writing. Let me tell you a little about my upbringing. My dad owned a beer joint. I would clean up the beer joint. I would fill the cooler, wash the glasses, sweep the floors, and carry out garbage. When I came home on leave from the Army, I would visit my dad at his beer joint. All his friends wanted to buy me a beer.

I would thank them, drink coke, and eat a hamburger or fried chicken with a salad. I drank a soft drink and ate French fries with them. We had a great time. Alcohol affects every part of your body. From your brain to your eyes, to your actions, to your language, to how you act, and to how you treat family and friends. The next day, you do not remember a thing. One of the saddest scenes I watched was a man so drunk that he was trying to go up seven steps. He got to the fourth step and passed out.

I have been all over the world. I have met a lot of people at parties who get drunk. They make an ass of themselves before a lot of people because they were so drunk and they did not know when to stop. The best thing is not ever to start drinking alcohol of any kind. This is the last thing I must tell you about. It is the most essential thing in your life, but only if you want to live as an old gentleman or lady.

What I am talking about is drugs. Not the medications your doctor prescribes to you and who runs many tests to see how each organ is doing. Your doctor is God's feelings to the world. Your doctor has spent many, many, many hours learning about you. Your doctor knows every organ in your body. He knows what each organ does to keep you alive for many years. Please thank your doctor each time you visit him for an exam for your pain, for which he prescribes medicine.

Thank your doctor for being there for any operation they perform on you. The doctor can add many, many years to your life. Always keep your appointment with your doctor. Follow their directions precisely as they tell you. I am not saying enough great things about doctors. Doctors spend many years in medical schools and many hours after school before they can practice medicine in their offices or hospitals.

Doctors have saved many lives because they take their jobs very seriously. Nurses work beside the doctor to keep you alive. Nurses are equally as important as doctors. The husband and wife need to have children and raise them to be good adult citizens.

Please, regardless of your age, DO NOT buy, sell, or take any drugs from the street. If you do not understand the street, I will tell you. Street drugs are sold to dumb people for money by people who do not give a damn about you except how much money they can get from you.

Please, please, please use your brain. Just think, why are they selling 'street drugs' to you? They do not like you. They don't care about you, they don't care about your parents, they don't care about your sister or brother or your parents. All they care about is money, money, money. The drug doctor's ``God" is the money" Can out of you for the drugs. The drug dealers have killed many young people and many business people.

Once you "do drugs" the first time, you have started down a road that will end in a graveyard. Many, many lives have been ruined because of drugs not being prescribed by doctors. I have been approached just to try one shot in the vein. I told them to go to hell. I have been contacted to take only one pill and see how you will feel. They paint a picture for you; take it, and you will be in heaven—a big fat joke. Just one shot or just one pill will send you to hell.

Many people die daily across America.

Just because of the drug kingpins, god is their money. Yes! They have a warm spot in hell waiting for them. Please, do not be led by a Hoop in the nose down the path of no return. "Think for yourself." "Think for yourself". I hope you

This world is beautiful, and every step taken has a meaning and a purpose. Just as the words we speak affects our lives and the lives of others, so do the actions that we are about to take today influence our lives and the lives of the people in the society. This is not confined to decisions that do not involve consumption of alcohol and use of drugs but it is the ability to make correct decisions that enable the person to live a satisfactory and healthy life.

Consider about the relationships you

value. Ethics are evident in how you handle other people that are close to you or people you work with. Maintaining these relationships with respect and love can produce a support system that assists one in dealing with life's issues. Always be surrounded by positive people and do not be that sort of person who bring down others. The relationships which are based on the respect and care are the only ones which are eternal and which make people happy.

Another vital component of a healthy schedule is education. One should always continue his education from formal education to the self-taught education, or through life experiences. Education enlightens you to make the right choices and unlocks opportunities that you probably never considered. Solicit desire and strive to comprehend the environment. This not only enlightens the human brain but also sharpens your personality and makes you a rather enjoyable company to have.

Exercises being important for heathy physical and mental living should be practiced on daily basis. Physically active has many benefits it increases your energy level, improve mood and reduce the risk of chronic diseases. It's not about getting a washboard abs or six pack abs, it is about training your body and getting it into a functional shape. Look for a sporting activity that you like, be it walking, dancing, sports or yoga among others. It is advised to perform this either daily, or in the least, make it one of the activities that you perform daily.

One's mental health is as vital as his or her physical health. Mental health is a crucial part of a person's health and includes behaviour and emotions, stress and coping, and self-care. Mindfulness and meditation help to bring peace in your mind and reduces the anxiety level. It is important always to consult mental health professionals, if it reaches to that, a point where you feel like, you cannot handle it anymore. It is not a sign of weakness to ask for help: on the contrary, it is a sign of wisdom and recognition of one's own weaknesses.

Another important pillar of a strong

health ecosystem is the intake of healthy diets. Remarkably, the fuel that is poured into a human body determines the intensity of energy, efficiency, and attitude towards life. Stress weight loss and a diet that comprises of fruits and vegetables, lean protein and whole grains.

Hydrogenated foods and sugars high fat or sugar products should be taken in moderation. Pay attention to your body and give it the nourishment that it requires through healthful foods that will not let you get tired quickly. Rest is unwanted at times but is a vital necessity in every person's life.

Quality sleep is the restoration and healing of the body, enhancement of thinking processes, and emotional condition. Make sure you are getting about seven to nine hours of sleep a day and try to stick to the same sleeping pattern. Establish relaxed pre-sleep time to reduce your activity and get ready for a good night's sleep.

Financial stability is another of the key components of a proper human life. Money management has the positive effect of relieving tension, and therefore results in less stress, while giving a person a feeling of financial security. Develop the capability to save for the future, develop personal budget and make proper decision related to spending and investing. Since there is financial security, it means that one does not have to be worrying all the time about the next meal.

Getting engaged in the community can

provide meaning and belonging to the clients. Dedicating your time and effort to others improves the recipients' well-being as well as brings personal satisfaction. Every help that you give to your fellow person, every kind word that you say to that person will go a long way in touching another life and making that life better.

There are many causes out there; you should find those you are interested in and contribute to them. It could be through volunteering, contributing financially or spreading the word through awareness this all goes a long way in helping. Without goals and an aim or purpose in achieving those goals life is mostly likely going to be perceived as meaningless.

Piggy on this, no matter what the targets

are about - work, study, self-improvement or wellbeing – it always helps to have something to look forward to. You want to set process goals and milestones, recognizing that goals are made up of small steps in accomplishing tasks. This roadmap is not merely or even mainly about the place, but the process and the changes that occur within you.

Thus, it can be seen that a positive attitude does saves a lot of energy and thus can have positive effect on the well-being. The world is not all rosy and that sometimes people are faced with hurdles and obstacles, the attitude towards these hurdles is paramount. Develop the coping strategies to be able to handle adverse situations and incidents without giving up.

Be optimistic and be thankful for the positive things that is happening in your life.

Positive attitude does not only contribute to the quality of your own life but also impacts on the quality of life of the people around the community. It is important to control and discipline oneself in order to stick to the set regular schedule. It is all about how to make decisions in accordance with something one prioritizes in his life and following it even when it is hard. Thus, self-discipline means learning how to successfully bring into practice the mechanisms of time and task management, avoiding distractions and vices that result in overall detrimental consequences.

As far as passive income is concerned, it is something that can be learned through practice coupled with hard work. Practicing mindfulness helps a person to relax, fight stress, and concentrate better due to the positive impact of meditation to the human body and mind. Spend some 10 to 20 minutes in the morning and before going to bed performing meditation, deep breath exercise, or simple being mindful. This can assist you in keeping the mind focused resulting in a stable and balanced approach to life.

Religious health, whatever concept a person may have, is also crucial. No matter if it is related to religion, self-contemplation, or revelation through nature, everyone should find a way to take care of their spiritual health. It is about the search for a purpose of living and having relation with other people or even with a higher power.

Hobbies are good for personal development, and creative activity serves an important function in one's life. Being creative can mean painting, putting pen to paper and writing, playing an instrument, tending a garden are rewarding. They are fun and help you to depart from the normal boring activities and at the same time can enable you discover new hidden abilities.

It is said and rightly so that every and each thing in life must be balanced. Try to prevent working and personal life from interfering and to achieve satisfactory degrees of occupational and social adjustment, self-development, and recreation. When fixing goals and objectives one has to be careful not to favor one area with goals at the disappearance of goals in other areas.

Living a balanced life avoids stress and in general, OSCE achieves a good quality of life. And, of course, the last nonverbal cue is appreciation appreciation of everything and everyone around you. Gratitude can be said to entail the identification and acknowledging of the favorable things in one's life. Sometimes they may be as uncomplicated as maintaining a gratitude list or a taking a few minutes at some point within a day to think about the things that you are grateful for. Gratitude brings attention to the good things one has, rather than the bad negatives or what one is lacking hence making one be more content.

Applying these principles in one's life can mean a healthier, happier, and more satisfying life. It's the process of selecting decisions with respect to the self and with regard to other people as well. This is a good place to start and the fact that you are here shows that you are willing to get up from the sick bed and set a routine that will make your life complete. The transformation does not happen in one day, but every little move that one makes towards the betterment of their health is a step to a better and fuller life.

Chapter 4: Maintaining the Physical and Mental Health

"Think for yourself" and take my advice, walk away from drugs, run away as fast as you can, and never look back. You can live to be 200 years old or live close to being an older man and an older woman. Sunday is the first day of the week, and the exercise starts on Sundays. Marked-down walks of fifty yards are the same for Monday, Tuesday, Wednesday, Thursday, Friday, and Saturday.

The second Sunday, start walking one hundred yards, write down, and go back. That is two hundred yards. Increase your walking by one hundred yards or one football field every Sunday for six months. You will be amazed at how great you feel and look. You are now on your way to two hundred years of age. "Do not overdo it. Next:

The next set of exercises is the most unique and remarkably effective. These exercises are done just before you fall asleep in bed. Once you are in bed, you do these exercises before you fall asleep.

Do these exercises, which will take about ten minutes or so. As you do them, the time will increase from five minutes to more. To start, all exercises will take about 5 minutes or less. As the reps increase, time will increase, and these will also begin in-bed exercises. Do these exercises, as I explained in bed.

1) Get in bed and lay on your back.

2) Your first exercise starts at your feet

A) Point your toes and feet forward at your head. This exercise stretches your calf and lower leg muscles, called "Gastrocnemius."

Count Ten thousand and one Ten thousand and Two Ten thousand and three Ten thousand and four Ten thousand and five Ten thousand and Six Ten thousand and Seven Ten thousand and eight Ten thousand and nine Ten thousand and ten.

Now

B) Next, Point your toes away from your head. This will stretch muscles on top of your lower legs. Count Ten thousand and one Ten thousand and Two Ten thousand and three Ten thousand and four Ten thousand and five Ten thousand and Six Ten thousand and Seven Ten thousand and eight Ten thousand and nine Ten thousand and ten. Do this for ten days. Get a calendar and make the day you start doing the exercises and how many reps you do. Count Ten thousand and one Ten thousand and Two Ten thousand and three Ten thousand and four Ten thousand and five. Ten thousand, Six Ten thousand, Seven Ten thousand, eight Ten thousand, and nine Ten Thousand and Ten.

This ten-day exercise tightens your upper legs and is called "quasigroup - 4 muscles in the upper leg.

Next;

Tighten your upper leg for a count of ten per night for 30 nights every night.

Next;

Tighten your butt muscle called Glutes for a count of ten for 30 nights every night.

Next;

Squeeze your testicles for a count of

ten for 30 days, men only.

Next;

Put the firsthand top of your thighs and push down on your thighs for a count of 10 for 30 days.

Next;

Put your first hand on the side thighs of your legs for a count of ten for 30 days.

Next;

Put your hand on your stomach and tighten your back muscles. Call Latinus close for a count of ten for 30 days.

Next;

Put the palms of your hands together for a count of ten for 30 days.

Next;

Put the palms of your hands together

about ten inches for a count of ten for 30 days.

Next;

With your palms together, raise your hands about ten inches away from your stomach, pointing to pushing your hands together for a count of ten for 30 days.

Next;

with your palms together, point your finger straight up toward the ceiling, pressing your hands together for a count of ten for 30 days.

Next;

Bring your hand down, make a bicep hard side with your right palms forward ideally, and bring your right palm toward your face and left palm away from your face for a count of 10 for 30 days. This exercise is for the upper arm biceps.

Next;

Hook your fingers with the back of your right hand towards your face for a count of ten.

Next;

Reverse your hook up your fingers with the back of your left hand toward your face for a count of ten slow for ten days.

Next;

Put your right fingers on the right side of your forehead and the upper part of your right head for a count of ten. Ten of them will push your head to your fingers.

Next;

Put your left fingers on the left side of your head for a count of ten and push toward your head.

Next;

Put all eight fingers on your raised head for a count of ten.

Next;

Put your first hand beside your body, palm down at your hips, and fist down on the mattress for a count of ten slow each day for ten days.

Next and last exercises.

With your right index finger and thumb, pinch your nose.

Next;

With your left palm put over your mouth, for a count five slow for 30 days.

Next;

Repeat the last exercise for a count

of ten.

Next

Repeat the First exercise for a count of 10 x 3. Done & Done.

We have such fundamental and integral components in our being that to ignore even one of them is a disservice to our very existence. In addition to physical activity and refraining from substances and activities that are damaging to the mind, mental health entails intentional healthy behaviors. Another preventive method is the usage of mindfulness.

Mindfulness means one is aware of what he or she does or think while doing it without any criticism. This practice can help in the reduction of stress, regulation of emotions and thus improve the general mental health of an individual. Start with mini-sessions of over breathing or body scan and then move to long sessions the longer your practice session becomes.

The third significant element is the positivity of the client's outlook. Positive attitude and positive thinking have been defined as having a very powerful effect on a person's well-being. First of all, one should try to fight negative fantasies and replace them with positive messages. Learn to concentrate on the positive aspects of your life, I matter how insignificant they are.

Give yourself a reason to be happy because every problem faced on the way is a small victory rather than a cause for dismay. Stay close to the people that speak well of you and motivate you. Their energy can be very invigorating, you get to be happy even when things are tough.

It is importance to sleep well for both body and the soul Sleep is a basic necessity to man.

To establish a regular pattern the person has to go to bed and get up at the same time every day including the weekends. Establish a correct set of behaviors before going to bed to let the organs know that you are getting ready for sleep. This could include reading a book, taking a warm bath or even the practicing of some forms of exercises like gentle stretching.

Interaction with electronic gadgets should be eliminated an hour to the time of the intended sleep since the light produced affects sleep. Make sure that the sleeping conditions are appropriate, there is no noise and no distractions around the house. Health is also determined by the kind of food you eat and the quality of food you take that greatly defines a person. A well-diversified diet consisting of adequate amounts of fruits, vegetables, whole-grain products, lean meats, fish, nuts, and low-fat dairy products can help meet all the body and brain's requirements.

Aim to drink adequate amounts of water at least a day, to help boost your water levels in the body. Do not consume large amounts of coffee and sweets because they cause the feeling of fatigue and shifts in temper. It is recommended that one includes foods such as fatty fish, nuts, and berries in their diet as they are helpful for the brain.

Belonging to groups or communities is one of the keys to good end frames of psychological wellbeing. Spending time alongside family and friends is also encouraged as is any social contact, that brings about happiness. Communicate with the team members; express yourself and the team members, and listen to others. Establishing support enhances companionship as this decreases loneliness and discourages the patient from feeling isolated.

Offer your time or participate in association, club, or any group activity of your preference. This part of community participation also plays a huge role in attainment of psychological satisfaction.

Engaging in activities of choice also enhances the mental health of a person, by so doing they get to follow hobbies and interests. Hobbies make you feel accomplished and are fun to do. Regardless of whether it is painting, gardening, the playing of an instrument, or cooking, spend time within those activities which make one contented. As we know hobbies can also act like an art form where a person can energize and forget his/her problems. In case, you have no hobbies, try learning new activities as a way of identifying your areas of interest.

One would agree with the idea that stress and its proper management are vital in maintaining a healthy mind. The sources of stress in one's life should be identified in order to work on a way of managing such stress. This might include having proper goals and objectives, the creation of small sub tasks and most importantly suing the proper time frames.

Use methods such as deep breathing, progressive muscle relaxation or visualization to calm your mind and body. Exercise can also be an effective method in stress management, because during exercise the body produces endorphins – substances which make people happier and less anxious.

If one fails to find a solution, one should not hesitate to get help from a professional. It is okay to seek help when one is in distress or has some issues regarding his or her mental health. Psychotherapists, counselors and psychologists are skilled in helping you manage life's difficulties and encouraging appropriate strategies for dealing with them. Psychotherapy makes it possible for one to express themselves and discover how they are feeling as well as make changes for the better.

It is important if you are displaying symptoms of a mental condition for example depression or anxiety you consult a doctor for proper medical attention. Goal setting as a way of achieving direction and purpose in life might be useful when the goals are attainable and arranged. It is recommended that you set process goals and sub- goals and make sure you practice goal posting and report your progress.

Work brings meaning or gives one an individual direction with a goal, this improves overall self-esteem and the feeling of achievement. Be sure, however, to know that it is perfectly alright to modify targets as well as the process is equally essential as the end result.

Religion can, for some, be inspirational and thus can provide source of hope to people when they are struggling. This does not have to be religion; it can mean belonging to nature, the universe, deeply personal creed, morality, and a lot more. There are spiritual ways that one could peruse and attain some sort of relief such as prayer, meditation or going for nature walks.

Mental strength is definitely important when it comes to one's ability to deal with life. A key component of living is that the good is always balance by the bad and thus resilience enables an individual to overcome the bad. Self-organization, self-positivity, and self-analysis. Be prepared to embrace change and seek assistance if and when required from other people.

Resilience means that one should not shame or blame himself or herself for his or her failures and defeats. Lastly, practice self-care regularly. Thus, self-care makes references to the process of investing time in the care of the body, mind and the spirit. This could include; enjoying a good book, taking a good bath, going for a walk, or even napping whenever you feel like it. Taking care of yourself is not a form of being self-indulgent; it is simply taking care of your health. Self-care is important and should not be overlooked, try to fit it in your schedule.

Thus, having such practices in one's life helps to be healthy physically and mentally and ensures a long, joyful, and meaningful existence. You must always bear in mind that your health is perhaps the single most important thing you can ever have, and thus, investing in it is the single best thing you can ever do.

Conclusion

Overall, this book has endeavored to serve as a manual for keeping up and improving physical and mental wellbeing using easily implementable strategies. The health-related topics addressed in each chapter are diverse, and the general view of a healthy, and long life has been offered.

Implementing the principles mentioned, starting with healthy habits and including physical and mental wellbeing principles, one can design a lasting lifestyle that includes the individual's quality of life goals.

Understanding the path to the definition of disease-free state: education and creating healthy lifestyles. Thus, it must be emphasized that the focus is on the concept of health as the lifelong journey and process to maintain or regain the healthy body and mind. If one is willing to make changes in their life, take baby steps every day and slowly learn how to make healthier choices, then their life can drastically change for the better.

Take into practice the recommendations by the authors and remain faithful to the intentions outlined in the book: You are designing your tomorrow. Choices you make today directly concern your health and your quality of life, yet all is not lost, in fact life can be absolutely fantastic. Let's keep it up, let's keep smiling, and please let's not forget the Mental Healthy Lifestyle.

The first chapter focuses on the feelings mentioned in the book and the position of the word of God as a map. The topic explains the authoritative origin of the Bible, the role of the Scripture and its role in relating to the world around and within us. The Chapter shows that recognizing existence by the framework of God's creation is a chief principle to live positively.

The next major concern is worship

and the honoring of God which is discussed in chapter 2. It explains how Christians are commanded to bow before God and to say that He is great. It explains the self-justification and the need to trust God and the penalty for not serving Him. It confirms the perception people held in thoseimes; that only if they devote their lives to the service of God, then they would be considered to have attained life's ultimate purpose.

Chapter three as a deep focus on the actual measures that have to be taken in order to set up a healthy schedule. Thus, the product contains a social notice prohibiting the use of alcohol and drugs because they are injurious to health. The chapter uses real-life examples and stories to explain why one should avoid taking substances and why a person should embrace a drug-free lifestyle. It also stresses on the importance of honoring medical recommendations as a way of keeping healthy.

The last clinical chapter is devoted to the description of physical exercises and mental health. It presents an extensive exercise regimen that is quite practical and adaptable to everyday use, stressing gradual advancement and repeatability. It also raises such topics as awareness, attitudes, sleep, diet, relations, and stress. It recommends the readers when to consult a doctor and when not and it urges people to be patient with themselves.

To be specific, all the chapters of the book present readers with an all-encompassing concept of health and wellness that takes into consideration the aspects of both the soul and the body as well as the mind. Regardless of the audience, it calls for preparation of adopting a healthy lifestyle ensuring that the reader is confident, strong, and empowered. Following the instructions given, the readers will be able to gain nicety and good health both in body and mind within the religious path.

Book Review Call

Thank you for taking the time to read "How to Live to Be 200 Years Old". I hope this book has inspired and equipped you with the tools to live a longer, healthier, and more fulfilling life. Now, I need your help to reach others who are starting their journey toward well-being. By leaving a review, you can guide someone toward discovering the benefits of building healthy routines, achieving mental and physical wellness, and understanding the power of self-reliance. If this book has been valuable to you, please consider sharing your thoughts. Your review could make all the difference to someone seeking a better life.

Made in the USA
Middletown, DE
04 November 2026

36545526R00057